BREAS

Everything you wanted to know but didn't know how or whom to ask

If you're a nursing mother, you need this book — to have a healthier and happier baby, and to have closer bonding that'll last you a lifetime. Mother's milk is the best and most natural food for a baby. Written exclusively for mothers by Dr. Sapna Samant, a medical expert, this book is a one-stop medical guide that'll help you to breast-feed successfully. From how to hold your baby while feeding, to how to generate more milk, from taking care of sore breasts to supplementing breast milk, here finally is a book that clears all the doubts your mind has voiced.

Books on Health & Cure

1. PREGNANCY: Everything you wanted to know but didn't know how or whom to ask
Dr.Monika Datta

2. YOU AND YOUR MEDICINES
Ranjit Roy Chaudhury

3. Speaking of CHILD CARE
Everything you wanted to know
Dr.Suraj Gupte

4. Speaking of SLEEPING PROBLEMS
Learning to Sleep Well Again
Dietrich Langen

5. Speaking of HEART ATTACKS
Early Recognition, Rehabilitation,
Prevention of Recurrence.
Carola Hal

6. Speaking of HIGH BLOOD PRESSURE
A Comprehensive Guide for Hypertensive
and Their Partners
Hanns P. Wolff, M.D.

7. CHILD CARE AND NUTRITION
Everything you wanted to know

Published by
Sterling Publishers Private Limited

BREAST-FEEDING

Everything you wanted to know but didn't know how or whom to ask

DR. SAPNA SAMANT

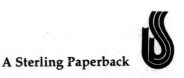

A Sterling Paperback

STERLING PAPERBACKS
An imprint of
Sterling Publishers (P) Ltd.
L-10, Green Park Extension, New Delhi-110016
Tel : 6191023, 6191784/85; Fax : 91-11-6190028
E-mail: ghai@nde.vsnl.net.in
Website : www.sterlingpublishers.com

*Breast-fedding: Everything you wanted to know but didnt know how
or whom to ask*
© 1998, Dr. Sapna Samant
ISBN 81 207 2043 1
Reprint 2000

Published by Sterling Publishers Pvt. Ltd., New Delhi-110016.
Laserset by Vikas Compographics, New Delhi-110029.
Printed at Shagun Offset, Safdarjung Enclave, Delhi-110029.
Cover design and illustrations by Piyush Garg

This book was not possible without
Supriya and Sadanand.
Thank you
Couldn't ask for more.

ACKNOWLEDGEMENTS

Shri P. Bhaskaran (Deputy Director, National Institute of Nutrition) for the weaning mixes.

Dr. R.K. Anand for his patience. For updating and for correcting all my mistakes.

Mrs Vaishakhi Bharucha for suggesting various improvements in the manuscript.

Dr. Sharadini Dahanukar for the ayurvedic galactogouges.

Dr. P.R. Deshpande for suggesting topics.

Dr. M.S. Kamath for giving me the right addresses.

Dr. Pramod Niphadkar for his input on allergy.

Dr. Rishma Pai for information on contraceptives.

And, last but not least, Dr. Manoj Bharucha for his encouragement and more encouragement.

CONTENTS

CONTENTS

1

Your Own Production Unit!

The breast has lots of tiny glands in which the milk is produced. These are connected to the nipple by small tubes called *ducts*. The ducts are arranged around the nipple like the spokes of a wheel.

The glands and ducts are supported by fat, blood vessels, and ligaments. These together are called the *connective tissue*.

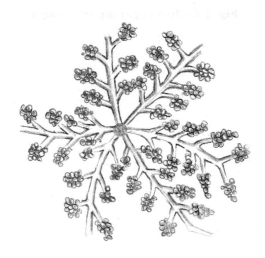

Fig. 1.1 : Lobes converging onto the nipple like spokes of a wheel.

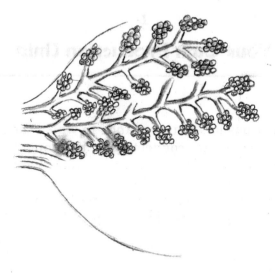

Fig. 1.2 : Ducts opening into nipple

2

Your Brain Is The Remote Control...

The brain secretes several hormones out of which two play an important role on breast-milk formation and secretion.

a) **Oxytocin:** It is secreted by the brain and causes ejection of milk.

b) **Prolactin:** It helps in the secretion of milk by the breast .

3

...And Your Baby Activates It

When your baby suckles, the message is carried to the brain which releases prolactin. As soon as the prolactin reaches the breast it stimulates the glands to produce milk. This is called *milk production reflex*.

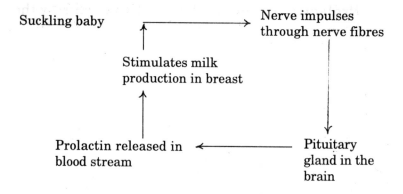

Suckling baby → Nerve impulses through nerve fibres

Stimulates milk production in breast

Prolactin released in ← Pituitary gland in the brain
blood stream

Fig. 3.1 : Milk producing reflex

At the same time, the brain also releases oxytocin which, when it reaches the breast, causes the milk to eject or come out. This is known as the *milk ejection reflex*. It is also called *milk let down*.

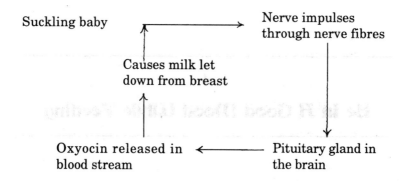

Fig. 3.2 : Milk Ejecting Reflex

You may feel pressure in your breasts just before a feed. That means the milk is starting to flow.

Ejection takes place within thirty seconds of the baby suckling. The opposite breast may also release a few drops of milk.

4

Be In A Good Mood While Feeding

Inhibition of milk let down can occur if you are in a state of shock or sudden anger or in pain.

Complete inhibition can occur if you are continuously under stress or are anxious. This hinders release of oxytocin and "let down" does not happen.

This leads to "drying up" and you often begin to doubt your ability to produce "enough" milk for the baby, increasing your anxiety which in turn inhibits 'let down'. So, always be in a good mood while feeding.

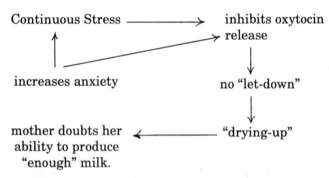

Fig. 4.1: Vicious Cycle Leading to "Let-Down" Inhibition

A baby's cry sometimes stimulates milk ejection. This is called ***conditioning***.

BE CONFIDENT AND DO NOT LISTEN TO ANY TALES.

Baby's Reactions

Every baby's attachment to its mother's breasts is inherent. Your baby too is attached to your breasts. It instinctively knows what to do when the breast is in its mouth.

If you touch a cheek of your newborn baby, it turns its head towards that side. If its lips are touched, the baby opens its mouth as if searching for a nipple to suckle. This is called **ROOTING REFLEX**.

The nipple has to touch the hard part of the baby's mouth above the tongue deep inside, enabling the infant to suckle.This helps in milk production and subsequent let down. The movement of the baby's mouth squeezes out the milk from the nipple. This is called the **SUCKLING REFLEX**.

Mother Nature's Gift

It is not as if the breasts produce a specific amount of milk everyday. The more you let your baby suckle, the more is the breast stimulated to produce milk. This is a natural process taking place in every single lactating mother. You should be confident of your individual capacity which is Mother Nature's gift. No amount of stories related to breast-feeding should disturb you. Only you can ensure complete nutrition for your child in the coming months.

7

Prepare Yourself For Breast-Feeding

You are expecting a baby. Or have just delivered.
You wonder. Will you be able to cope?
YES!
You have decided to breast-feed. You are on the right track.
Your body has also prepared itself for the act.
Prepare your nipples for feeding.

Types of Nipples

To know which type of nipples you have, stand against a mirror and look at the profile of both the breasts.
There are four types of nipples:

1) Average.
2) Short/ Flat
3) Inverted/ Retracted
4) Long.

If the nipples are of average size, they will appear like this:

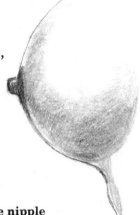

Fig. 7.1 : Average nipple

9

If the nipples are short or flat they will appear like this:

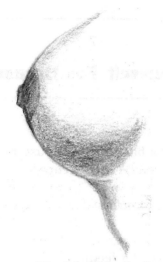

Fig. 7.2 : Flat nipple

Inverted or retracted nipples appear like this:

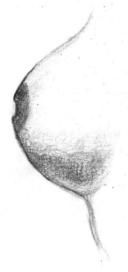

Fig. 7.3 : Inverted/retracted nipple

Long nipples look like this:

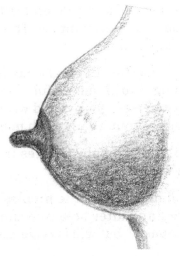

Fig. 7.4 : Long Nipple

Short or retracted nipples are no cause for worry. You can prepare each type of nipple in the following way.

Average Nipples

Repeatedly pull the nipples out without hurting, daily for a dozen times each. This should generally be done during the last month of pregnancy.

Short / Flat Nipples

Initially, the pulling out may be difficult as the nipple may slip between the fingers. Hold the nipple between the thumb and first two fingers and gently pull it out several times without hurting or getting tired. This should be done for more than a month. Patience will pay and the flat nipples will protract (come out).

Inverted / Retracted Nipples

Pulling out these nipples may again cause difficulty. Some nipples are non-protractile because they are attached by strands of tissue to the glands. But this is a

11

rare occurrence. Trying to pull out inverted nipples like flat nipples does help. The nipple protracts a short way because it is generally a short nipple. This will be pulled out when the infant sucks.

A truly non-protractile nipple also needs to be worked on if breast-feeding is to be successful. You may continue the pulling out exercises (gently) and wear nipple shells inside your brassiere from the seventh month onwards.

Understand that the baby suckles from the breast and not just the nipples.

Inverted and non-protractile nipples may improve during pregnancy and after breast-feeding is initiated. They may not "pop-out" but will become more protractile.

Let the baby suckle in a good position, and let it suckle early before the breasts become full.

If the baby does not take the breast properly, express the milk and feed by cup or spoon. Meanwhile, try to get the baby to take the breast properly.

When your baby sucks, the nipples will be stretched and pulled, sometimes chewed.

By preparing your nipples you can avoid soreness.

> THE ABILITY TO FEED DOES NOT DEPEND UPON THE SIZE AND SHAPE OF THE BREAST.

You may be told that breast-feeding is a problem-ridden job, not at all easy. You may have to listen to all kinds of tales. Don't get anxious or stressed.

Childbirth is an overwhelming experience.

Mild depression, irritability, weepiness, dullness, slowness, etc., are what 99 per cent women suffer from after the third or fourth day of delivery. These are called *maternity blues* or *baby blues*.

If your child is fussy and cries a lot you may worry about how you will be able to look after a fragile, helpless infant. You may doubt your ability to feed the infant.

Mentally prepare yourself for such blues, unpleasant tales, initial feeding problems, adjustments, etc.

Feed Successfully and It is Your Triumph.

To relax yourself you can listen to your favourite music, meditate or visit the local place of worship if it helps you.

One girl I know was repeatedly told by her relatives that her milk would dry by the second month. It did. All she heard after that was "We told you so." Her milk stopped because she believed her relatives rather than her own ability to secrete well.

8

Starting Breast-Feeding

Now you know where your milk comes from and how it is controlled.

You are mentally and physically prepared.

The next question on your lips is...

When to Give the First Feed?

It is never to soon for your first feed. Hold the baby near the naked breast after delivery, fondle it, cuddle it. These are important components of the "first feed". The baby may try to get hold of the nipple with its mouth. If it succeeds let it suckle.

The hospital or nursing home where you deliver will invariably keep the baby in the nursery after it has been weighed and cleaned. According to them, you will be too exhausted to hold the baby, forget feeding it. (Who are they to decide?)

Insist on having your baby back and hold it to your breast. It will start sucking on its own.

What you will feel overcomes all exhaustion. There aren't enough words to describe the joy!

The first feed will be a straw-coloured fluid—the *colostrum.* It is absolutely necessary for the baby. As you continue feeding, the colostrum will change to milk after a few days. Till then the colostrum is sufficient nutrition for the infant.

Never discard the first fluid from the breast.

How Often Should You Feed?

There is no fixed pattern of feeds. Every baby is an individual. It may be fussy and demanding or may have a quiet and undemanding temperament. Some babies have a small stomach capacity and require a feed every hour. Others have a larger stomach capacity and may be satisfied with fewer feeds.

An infant may not feel very hungry for a day or two after its birth. From the third or fourth day onwards, its demands increase. After the first week, your baby will establish its own routine for feeds and you have to give milk accordingly.

There is no such thing as too many feeds or too few feeds. A baby may take up to 10-15 feeds per day depending on how hungry it feels. During the night too a baby requires feeding.

The only fixed norm in the pattern of feeding is that MILK SHOULD BE FED ON DEMAND, i.e., there should be unrestricted feeding.

You may be advised to feed the baby every 3 hours or 4 hours or according to the clock. This pattern is supposed to inculcate disciplined habits in infants.

Infants do not need any such form of "discipline" regarding feeds.

In fact, it may keep the infant hungry, and hunger makes it cranky and fussy, with reduced growth.

Thus fixed timings is a wrong concept.

So the demand pattern should be followed.

How Long Should You Feed

There is no fixed pattern. Every baby will suckle as much milk as it wants and then stop. If you feed correctly the baby will empty 90 percent of the feed in the first 4-5 minutes itself. It is important to check your position. If it is uncomfortable or is being suffocated then the baby will stop suckling.

You will often be told that if the baby suckles for long the nipples become sore. (Haven't a lot of people told you this?)

Soreness will occur only if the feeding position is wrong, leaving the baby dissatisfied.

Very short feeds can also leave the baby dissatisfied (as it has not taken the hindmilk) and the breasts get engorged as they have not been emptied.

I am sure you have met a mother who cooed about how good her baby was. It never demanded feeds, made no fuss about wanting more and accepted when feeds were given.

Did she tell you that your demanding baby needed to be disciplined?

Well, you can ask her if she eats when hungry or starves herself till it is the right time.

Your little baby understands the needs of its stomach. Give as often as it wants and as long as it takes.

There may be something wrong with a baby which never demands feeds and is lethargic and placid.

Look after your nipples.
No extra care necessary.
A clean bath is sufficient.
Secreting milk itself is like a cleansing process.
Never use spirit to clean the nipples at any time.
Spirit is an alcohol and alcohols dry the skin.
Never use antiseptics or artificial cleansing agents.

Positions in which You can Feed

A comfortable position is a must.

a) This ensures you are not anxious or tense, helping in stimulating secretion.

b) This also ensures that the nipple and the areola are within reach of your infant's mouth and that it can suckle easily without too much effort.

c) Due to awkward positioning, the breast may fall on your infant's face, covering the nostrils and suffocating it. This makes the baby leave the breast to breathe by its mouth. It may also start crying, and you become tense and anxious, which in turn reduces milk production and secretion.

d) If breast-feeding gives you pain in the nipples, you are not seated in the correct position. The most common cause of sore nipples is odd positioning.

A baby may have been offered the bottle at the maternity home, while waiting for the breast-milk to come in. When given the breast, such a baby will pull at the nipple like it is a rubber teat, causing soreness.

OFFER THE WHOLE BREAST. NOT JUST THE NIPPLE.

Position for Breast-feeding

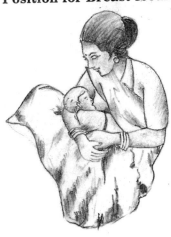

Positions for Breast-feeding

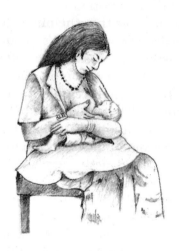

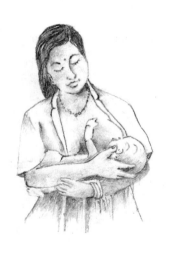

Positions for Breast-feeding

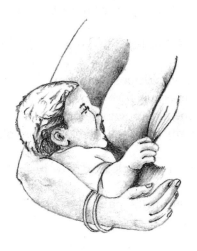

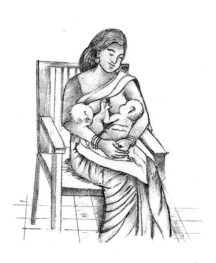

While feeding check that:
1) The baby faces you.
2) The baby has taken in the nipple, the whole areola, and its chin is touching the breast.
3) It makes satisfied swallowing sounds with deep, slow sucks.

This shows that the baby is in a good position and is feeding correctly.

If the baby is in an odd position then
1) The baby does not face you.
2) The chin doesn't touch the breast.
3) It suckles only at the nipple and most of the areola is seen.
4) The sucks are quick and the baby fusses while feeding.
5) You may feel nipple pain.

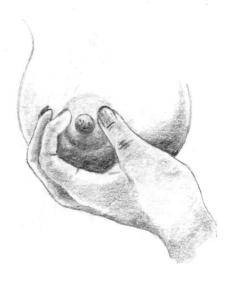

Fig. 8.1 Offering only nipple

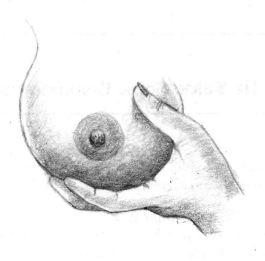

Fig. 8.2 Offering whole breast

Burping after Feeds

If you breast-feed, there is less chance of air being swallowed along with the milk. A bottle fed baby swallows much more air. Put the baby across the shoulder and gently pat on the back. A small amount of milk (mostly curdled) may come out along with air. This is called regurgitation and is unimportant.

Let Us Solve Some Common Problems

Each one of you will have some query or doubt. I will try to answer the most common ones.

Why do Breasts Engorge?
Very commonly, your breasts are engorged on the third or fourth day when more milk comes in.

This condition maybe painful, causing tender breasts. There may also be a touch of fever.

Engorgement of breasts occurs because initially,

a) The breasts are congested by blood and tissue fluid.
b) There is excessive production of milk which suddenly fills the breasts.

The blood and tissue fluid reduce spontaneously and the milk production is soon regulated according to the baby's demands.

The best way to relieve this engorgement is to put the infant to the breast frequently and allow it to suckle. This way the breasts are emptied of milk. Otherwise, the milk could be expressed out.

The breasts become softer and more pliable. There is no need to worry that this form of emptying will fill the breasts with excessive milk. The breasts automatically adjust to the demands of the baby.

If the breasts are not emptied by suckling or expression, there are high chances of the milk within becoming infected leading to a condition called *breast abscess.*

How to Treat Sore Nipples

You may get sore nipples in the first week as the baby chews and pulls them. There is a solution.

First let us look at the causes.
The causes of sore nipples are:

1) Faulty positioning
2) Inverted nipples
3) Engorged breasts
4) Faulty suckling

Sore nipples are often only slightly reddish, sometimes having small cracks and leaks of blood. They are extremely painful.

Prevention is better than cure. The conditions causing sore nipples should be avoided. If, in spite of avoidance, sore nipples begin to develop then:

a) Try changing the nursing position. This way the parts of the nipple subjected to pulling and chewing are changed.
b) Rub the last few drops of milk (hindmilk after feeds) on the nipples. Breast-milk has anti-infective properties.

Never use spirit, tincture iodine, medicated ointments or alcohol preparations on the sore nipples as they damage the skin more.

c) Give short, frequent feeds to the infant. This way the breast is emptied even though the act is very painful. Maximum rest to the nipple is not the solution. Give the unaffected or least affected breast to the infant. Then change over to the sore breast.
d) Manual expression or emptying of the breast after the infant has been fed can be done. This helps in preventing abscess formation and also exercises the nipples.

f) After the infant finishes feeding, it will pull at the nipple while withdrawing it's mouth. This aggravates the soreness. To prevent this put a finger in the infant's mouth and disengage the nipple slowly from the infant's mouth.

g) If the nipple is very sore then temporarily discontinue feeding on that side. The milk should be expressed and fed to the baby by katori/wati or spoon. It can also be stored.

Sore nipples can be easily cured. Lots of patience, encouragement from others and the will to continue breast-feeding is needed. Don't use it as an excuse to stop feeding the baby and put it on the bottle.

In spite of treatment, sometimes sore nipples persist. This could be because:

a) The baby has an infection in its mouth which needs to be cured. It is called *thrush* and is usually occurs during the third week, if it happens at all.

b) There is a deep crack or fissure in the nipple itself which does not heal with conventional treatment and may need antiseptics or antibiotics.

c) Allergic reactions of the nipple to an ointment or the detergent used to wash the brassieres or irritability caused by the pads in a brassiere.

All the above three conditions are curable but need individual attention, hence the family doctor should be consulted if there is any doubt.

Breast-feeding may not be possible in these conditions but milk expression should be done. This way feeding can be resumed immediately after the soreness is cured.

What is a Milk Blister?
This condition is rare. One sees a small white blister on the nipple. This is because the milk gets under the superficial layers of the skin. Nursing should be continued. The blister will disappear by itself.

Preventing Breast Abscess

Infection within the breast or its inflammation is pretty common. One of the causes for this is stagnation of the milk within the breast.

During lactation, the breasts need to be emptied of milk, either by the suckling infant or by expression. Failure to do so causes stagnation of milk in the breasts, leading to engorgement. The breasts become tense and tender due to inflammation. An inflamed breast is an invitation to infection. Eventually, there is pus formation within the breast which can be cured by antibiotics and drainage.

Prevention of abscess is done only by emptying the breast.

Leaking is so Embarrassing!

This is a common problem. The staining of clothes and the foul smell are really embarrassing in public.

It can occur at the slightest cry of your baby, cloth rubbing against the nipple, approach of feeding time, etc.

Wear cloth, absorbent tissue or cotton in your bra. Change them often. Marketed pads are also available for putting in the bras.

What will you do if it occurs in the other breast while baby is feeding on one? Press it like a doorbell or you could collect the milk in a cup to be fed later.

As lactation continues, leaking reduces.

Is it Normal for the Baby to Demand Feeds at Night? Should You Feed it?

It is perfectly normal to demand feeds at night. They should NEVER BE DENIED. Initially, the infant will demand feeds constantly, even at night. These reduce as time progresses.

If you have fed your baby well during the day then it might not ask for feeds at night. Only some infants are "night timers" and tend to demand feeds at night.

Your Milk is Not Enough!

Isn't that what everyone keeps telling you? You are going to secrete milk according to the status of your body as well as the demands made by the baby.

Secretion of milk is a cascade.

Suckling by baby

↓

More prolactin formation

↓

More milk produced

↓

Sufficient for the baby.

If you think your milk is less and start on top feeds, then the production will automatically reduce as the baby stops sucking.

Weigh your child on the same scale over a period of several weeks to check gain of weight. Just a constantly crying and hungry baby is not proof enough of insufficient milk.

A satisfied and healthy baby gains a minimum of 125 gms per week.

Over a month it should gain from 1/2 to 1 kilo.

Helping mothers to breast-feed. Indian adaptation by R. K. Anand.

Mark the baby's weight on the growth chart. If it is following the reference curve the baby is getting enough milk. If the baby's weight is lower and does not follow the reference curve, don't rush to give supplements or top feeds.   Think.

★ Are you feeding the baby as and when it demands milk?

★ Are you making the feeds short and not letting the baby suckle for as long as it wants?

★ Check the suckling position. The baby may be fussing because it is taking in only the nipple.

★ You may not have understood the wisdom behind breast-feeding and may have started supplements too early. They are unsuitable for the child as it is unable to properly digest them and they do not aid growth. Besides, your breast-milk production will reduce as you are not getting enough stimulus.

Some babies fall asleep in the middle of a feed. Gently stroke the cheek to wake it up.

Do not swaddle the baby in many clothes while feeding. It will make the baby uncomfortable.

The baby may be ill and needs to be shown to a doctor.

Only 1per cent mothers among you will genuinely have low milk production. But that does not mean that they should completely stop breast-feeding.

Give your own milk and to ensure that the infant receives human milk only, let a surrogate mother or a wet nurse feed the child. Give her a complete health check-up first. She should have genuine affection for the child. This method ensures complete nutrition to the infant.

Pity that it is widely unaccepted in almost all classes of our society though there are many instances of surrogate feeding in Indian mythology e.g. Yashodara feeding the baby Lord Krishna.

You can also try several galactogogues., i.e. drugs and foods which may increase your milk production. Consult a doctor who is well informed about medication and breast-feeding.

If supplements (i.e. only if your doctor feels they are necessary. You must not decide on your own) need to be given, liquid milk is preferred to powder milk.

Up to 4 months of age 2 parts of pure cow's milk + 1 part boiled and cooled water.

After 4 months of age
Undiluted cow's milk.
Add a teaspoon of sugar to 120 ml (4 oz) of the feed.

If pure buffalo's milk has to be used, please remove the cream before preparing the feed.

Give about 5 feeds every 4 hours.
Start with 30 ml (1oz) per kilo body weight per feed.
Do not give the night feed. Instead, breast-feed.

If you do use powder milk, take the following proportion:
1 level measure of powder milk : 30 ml (1 oz) of boiled cooled water.

Helping mothers to breast-feed. Indian adaptation R. K. Anand.

Preferably avoid all these preparations.
It is important that you don't give up on yourself. You must try and improve your milk production.
Never use the bottle when feeding these supplements. Always use a spoon or feeding cup.

My Milk has Stopped Coming!
When you doubt your ability to produce enough milk and also hear various stories about "drying of milk", you will subconsciously look for such signs within yourself.

Frequent feeds is the trick here. You have the potential to produce enough milk and this can be exploited. Don't rush to get the bottle-feeding paraphernalia. Be confident.

My Milk is Too Thin!
Milk produced by humans is thin. It is slightly watery, with a tinge of blue. Don't try to compare it to animal milk. You are not a cow or a buffalo. Though thin, human milk is perfect nutrition for your baby.

My Baby Keeps Crying!

This plaint I have heard too often. I know it worries you too.

Your baby could be crying because:

1) It is fussy and cranky by nature—this you can't help.
2) It has passed urine or stools which you can clean.
3) The baby is not getting enough milk. Either you have cut the feeds and feeding time due to which the baby suffers, or, the baby is not getting enough hindmilk which is rich in fat and supplies most of its energy needs. Or, there could be other problems. (See "My milk is not enough")
4) It has colic. This I shall explain later.

A Quiet Baby is a Good Baby

Not necessarily. Some babies never demand feeds, some refuse to suckle. It may have a cold or may be suffocated by the breast while feeding. Keep tabs on the weight. If it is increasing as required, then there isn't much cause for worry. If not, then your baby needs to be seen by it's doctor. Look for rational reasons and you will find them.

My Periods Have Not Yet Restarted/My Periods are Irregular.

Oestrogen and progesterone are two hormones present in high quantities during pregnancy. After the baby is born, the placenta comes out of the uterus. This is a major source of oestrogen and progesterone secretion. Thus, there is a sudden drop in the levels of these two hormones. At the same time the mother starts lactation. Lactation (secretion and feeding of milk) prevents ovulation, hence menstruation. So, if you are lactating, then you may not get your periods for sometime.

Your body, meanwhile, is slowly returning to its pre-pregnancy state. The uterus reduces in size, the ovaries start producing oestrogen and progesterone in small quantities. When the levels are high enough to stimulate ovulation, menstruation will take place.

The time of the first period after delivery varies in every individual. Some women may start menstruating within 6-8 weeks post-pregnancy. Periods may be regular or irregular. It is not abnormal to have irregular periods till you are feeding.

Breast-feeding does help in child spacing by prolonging menstruation. But it is not completely foolproof.

You may experience pain in the uterus during feeding. This is because the muscles in the uterus are contracting. It is of no consequence.

Remember

It is your right to put your baby to the breast immediately after delivery and start feeding there itself.

The more your baby suckles at the breast, the more milk is produced.

Demand feeding pattern should be followed during the day and at night.

Duration of each feed should be for as long as the baby suckles.

Good positioning and offering enough breast ensures proper feeding

---

10

ꓮ Feeding Mother's Diet

Isn't it a miracle that for all the various foods you eat, you produce this liquid with perfectly balanced nutrients which is complete nourishment for your child? An infant doesn't have to have different foods to satisfy its hunger and requirements, for a mother's milk is just perfect.

Your Nutritional Requirements
Every mother, rich or poor, has enough capacity to produce breast milk for her child unless she is grossly malnourished.

Your body has stored fat during pregnancy. It is used as energy for milk production. Even a so-called undernourished woman has energy stores to suffice her for the initial 4-6 months of lactation.

Yet, certain requirements should be fulfilled.

What are the Correct Foods to be Eaten by a Lactating Mother?
As mentioned before, you can make milk out of any food. A mother should have enough food. Seasonal fish, fruits and raw vegetables should be included in the diet.

Rice, dal, chappatis, fish, meat, all kinds of vegetables, fruits, curries should be consumed. In some Indian families, ghee, almonds, raisins, sultanas, etc., are added specially to a mother's meal. They help in building subcutaneous fat deposits. If you have a tendency towards obesity, these foods should be consumed with a little precaution. Every day, wholesome home-cooked meals are the best food for a lactating mother. You must drink enough water to quench your thirst. Spices and condiments can be consumed but sparingly.

What are the Sources of Vitamins and Minerals?
VITAMIN A: This is present in green leafy vegetables, carrots, eggs, mangoes, milk and milk products, meat, fish. It promotes growth and resistance to infection.

VITAMIN B_1: It is found in rice, peas, beans, oatmeal, meat, outer layer of cereal grains, peanuts, wheat, wholesome bread, fruits and fresh vegetables. The richest source is parboiled *(poha)* and unpolished rice. Rice bran is cooked and the water is added to everyday food if polished rice is eaten.

VITAMIN B_2: It is available through liver, kidney, meat, vegetables, egg and milk.

VITAMIN B_3: It is found in yeast, wheat, peanuts, milk, cereals, liver and meat.

VITAMIN B_6: It is found in milk and meat, cereals, legumes and yeast.

VITAMIN B_{12}: It is commonly found in non-vegetarian foods. Meat, liver, kidney, oysters, fish, egg yolk are rich in vitamin B_{12}. Vegetarians can obtain vitamin B_{12} from milk, milk products, legumes and nodules of root vegetables (radish, beet, etc.).

NIACIN: It is found in large quantities in rice, liver, eggs, milk, lean meat and potatoes.

FOLIC ACID: It is found in abundance in green vegetables, liver and yeast. Moderate amounts are found in eggs, meat, fish and dairy foods. Prolonged boiling of food destroys the folic acid content.

VITAMIN C: Fruits are a major source of this vitamin. It is also found in potatoes and fresh green vegetables. Citrus fruits and tomatoes should be consumed.

VITAMIN D: This is produced naturally in the skin on exposure to sunlight. About 20 minutes of daily morning sunlight should suffice in helping form vitamin D. In a sunny country like India, deficiency of this vitamin should not be seen. Yet, it is common. Dietary sources are fish, liver oils, butter, milk and yolk of egg.

VITAMIN E: It is present in soya bean, wheat and germ rice oil and the green leaves of lettuce.

The important minerals required are:

CALCIUM: Milk and milk products are the richest source of calcium. Green leafy vegetables, rice, ragi (millet) and cereals are also rich in calcium. Unfortunately, the average Indian diet overall has a poor content of calcium which can be used by the body. Hence, all lactating mothers need supplementation.

Iron: An Indian diet has an adequate amount of iron content. Yet, dietary deficiency is so common. Green vegetables, peas, beans, bananas, spinach, cereals, egg yolk, meat and liver are sources of iron. Iron is better absorbed by the body from animal foods than from vegetable foods. Milk and milk products are a good source of iron.

Did you know that you have two sources of natural irons right in your kitchen?

The iron cooking utensils and jaggery (*gur*)! Use one to cook and make chappatis. Use the other instead of sugar. The entire family can utilise these sources.

Eating a tiny ball of gur mixed with peanut powder or mashed peanuts is also an effective way of fighting dietary deficiency in iron, fats, carbohydrates and proteins.

Other minerals--ZINC, COPPER, MAGNESIUM, MANGANESE, IODINE, FLUORINE, etc.--known as trace elements are also a necessary part of a lactating mothers diet. These trace elements are found in green vegetables, milk and milk products, meat, fish, liver, kidney, eggs, etc.

Dietary Deficiencies and Their Effects

PROTEINS: While producing milk the body has the capacity to reach into its protein stores if diet is lacking in proteins. If protein deficiency is present, the mother will suffer from lethargy and generalised malnutrition. Similarly, lack of proteins will be passed through the milk to the child who will suffer from specific protein energy malnutrition.

FATS: Human milk is very rich in fats. The mother has also stored sufficient amount of fat antenatally. Fat is essential for the development of your infant's nervous system, i.e. brain and nerves, etc. You also need it as a source of energy. Deficiency in fat content will cause a gradual drop in milk production and underdevelopment of the infant's nervous system.

SUGARS: These are glucose, lactose, fructose starch, etc. The lactating mother needs these to maintain the various processes taking place within her body, i.e., for her metabolism. The child needs them for its metabolism and also as a source of energy. Through milk only the sugar lactose is available which is sufficient for the infant's metabolism and energy needs if present in sufficient amount in milk.

VITAMIN A: If a lactating mother has vitamin A deficiency, she rarely has any problems. The deficiency is passed on through reduced content in milk to the infant. It causes night blindness, white spots on the conjunctiva and dry eye. There may also be dry skin, diarrhoea and complete blindness.

The various vitamins B are together called the *B complex* group. They have a range of functions, right from helping in metabolism, to maintaining skin and other tissues, forming red blood cells, helping in digestion, strengthening nerves, etc.

VITAMIN B$_1$: Deficiency in infants—this causes convulsions(fits), vomiting, anorexia, green stools and sudden death. In adults it causes loss of body weight, apathy, irritability, depression.

VITAMIN B$_2$: Deficiency causes inflammation of mouth and tongue, reddened, shiny, chapped lips, burning feet, conjunctivitis, reduced vision.

VITAMIN B$_3$: There is headache, vomiting, sleepiness, nausea, tingling numbness, lethargy, malaise.

VITAMIN B$_6$: Deficiency causes failure to gain weight, irritability, twitching, convulsions. In adults, it may cause skin lesions, convulsions and mental changes.

VITAMIN B$_{12}$: Anaemia is seen in this deficiency. It helps in the uptake of folic acid, another necessary vitamin. Hence, B$_{12}$ deficiency may also cause folate deficiency which further aggravates anaemia.

NIACIN: In adults as well as children, niacin deficiency causes inflammation and pigmentation of skin, anorexia, lethargy, inflammation of tongue, diarrhoea and anaemia.

FOLIC ACID: This is required in the formation of various necessary chemicals within the body. Deficiency causes anaemia. As it is a nerve tonic, lack of folic acid may lead to mild confusional states. If there is folic acid deficiency during pregnancy, it causes defective spinal cord formation in the foetus.

VITAMIN C: It helps in the formation of cartilage, bone, teeth, healing of wounds, formation of haemoglobin and red blood cells. In adults there are blood clots in the skin, bleeding in the tissues, bleeding spongy gums and anaemia. Similar changes may be seen in the gums and skin of infants. There is also loss of appetite, listlessness, bleeding within the bones.

VITAMIN D: This vitamin is necessary for the incorporation of calcium in the bones. Deficiency causes a specific condition in infants called rickets. In this there is softening of bones leading to deformation.

CALCIUM: Apart from vitamin D deficiency, which causes calcium deficiency, dietary lack of calcium also leads to various conditions. In the mother an already present calcium deficiency (so common in India) is aggravated in pregnancy and lactation. It may lead to adult rickets known as *ostoemalacia*. In infants it causes weakening of the heart, bones and teeth. There is improper functioning of a hormonal gland called the *parathyroid*. Specific lack of calcium leads to convulsions.

Iron: This element is necessary for the formation of haemoglobin, which is an important component of blood. Iron deficiency causes anaemia. Presence of vitamin C helps in the absorption of iron.

The nutritional needs of a baby start in the womb. It is thus important for a mother to eat the correct foods during pregnancy itself and continue the proper diet when she is lactating.

It is also clear that the various necessary elements and foods complement each others functioning, so all should be included in the diet.

You must Avoid...

Fried foods dripping with oil, too much sugar, salt, tea and coffee. Smoking, alcohol and hard drugs should be completely avoided.

Galactogogues/Foods which may Help in Increasing Milk Production.

They have been passed on for generations, are nutritionally rich and completely harmless.

Some are:
    rice/ rawa porridge
    methi laddoos
    edible gum (dink) laddoos
    chicken soup
    crab soup
    herb teas
    methi kheer
    liver
    sweet shira prepared in ghee
    paya soup, etc.

11

Cosmetic Changes And Breast-Feeding

The Shape of the Breast may Change

In a first pregnancy the whole breast increases in size. The glandular tissue also increases in preparation for feeding.

To support the glands, the connective tissue also increases.

The breasts become heavier and enlarged and sensitive to touch.

The nipple and areola both turn dark in colour. This is more in dark-skinned people.

The skin of the breasts is stretched and thinned giving rise to whitish streaks commonly called *stretch marks*. The ligaments within the breast tissue are also stretched.

The blood supply of the breasts also increases and there may appear dilated bluish veins under the breast skin.

A thin straw-coloured fluid may be secreted from the breasts.

All these changes indicate activation of the breasts and may take place from the second month of pregnancy.

If not adequately supported, the breasts tend to become pendulous (hang down). This tendency increases with subsequent pregnancies.

Breast-Supporting Brassieres and other Garments
Unsupported breasts almost always turn pendulous in shape. You should wear proper fitting nursing bras. Similarly, other housegowns and nighties are also available. The saree blouse or choli is one such piece of clothing. Its tight fit gives support to the breasts and the front opening offers convenience during feeding.

Are there Any Exercises You can do to Help Maintain the Shape?
Yes there are.
These exercises are aimed at tightening the breast ligaments and developing the chest muscles on which the breasts lie.

a) Push-ups help in strengthening the chest muscles. Start with a minimum of 5 push ups daily and gradually increase up to 25 or more.
b) Alternately, stand at arms, length to a wall with both palms flat on the wall. Push the upper half of the body towards the wall, at the same time push at the wall with both palms. Make sure the feet are in their original position. Get back at arms length after a count of 10. Do this about 20 times twice daily.

Fig. 11.1

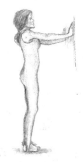

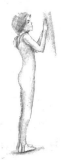

Arms against
the wall

Pushing wall Feet
firmly on ground

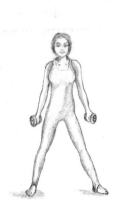 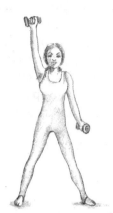 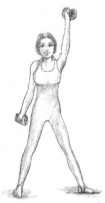

| Hands gripping weights | Arm carrying weight, straight up | Opposite arm with weight, straight up |

c) Sit crossed-legged with a spine straight or stand absolutely erect. Take both hands behind the neck and lock the first two fingers of each hand in a grip. Pulling at the grip yet keeping the fingers locked, lift both arms completely above the neck. Keeping the pull on the fingers, bring the arms down with the hands behind the neck. Relax. Tighten the grip again to repeat the motion 10 times. Do it twice daily.

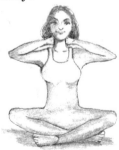 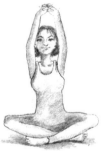

Hands locked behind neck

Arms straight up. Fingers locked.

Spine erect at all times

d) Take two equal weights (heavy books or dumb-bells) in one hand each. Lift one arm completely and straight above the head. Hold for a count of 5. Bring it down. Now lift the other arm holding the weight. Keep for a count of 5. Bring it down. Repeat action alternately with both arms holding weights. Increase gradually from a minimum count of 5 to 25.

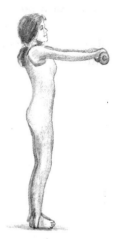

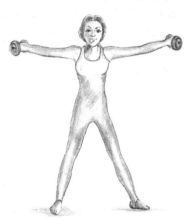

Arms with weight, straight ahead— view from side

Arms with weights, straight in line with shoulders, perpendicular to ground. Stand on toes—view from front.

Spine erect at all times

e) Holding the weights in each hand, stretch both arms completely in front of the chest. Simultaneously, take both arms away from each other till they are stretched sideways and perpendicular to the body. Stand on the toes at the same time. Slowly bring them back in front of the chest, stretched and parallel to the ground. Get back on your feet. Repeat the action fast, gradually increasing from 10 to 50 times. One has to stand erect throughout.

These exercises will show results over a period of time, depending upon the regularity with which you perform. Consult your doctor before you start them. Wear a bra at all times.

Control Your Figure—Breast-feed

Having eaten the "correct foods" during pregnancy, losing weight during lactation is easy. The act of breast feeding utilises the fat deposits on your body as a source of energy. This results in loss of body fat and a gradual return to original body weight. In fact, if you are feeding, you will lose weight faster than a mother who is not feeding.

12

Sex, Contraception And Breast-Feeding

Culturally, in our society, sex is taboo for the traditional 40 days rest period. This invariably occurs because the woman is at her parents house and the husband in his house.

Otherwise, there is no such taboo on sex.

In fact, you will have heightened interest in sex.

You may find breast-feeding sexually stimulating. This is because:

1) Breast stroking takes place during breast-feeding and can also occur in sexual foreplay.
2) Nipple erection occurs with or without nipple stimulation in sexual activity and feeding.
3) Contractions of the uterus occur in suckling and sexual arousal, even anticipation of sex.
4) Let down can be stimulated by sexual excitement also.

Emotionally, breast-feeding and sexual activity are similar in the feelings they arouse. Many of you will thus feel uninhibited about sexual activity.

Contraception

Lactation prolongs the return of menses as ovulation is suppressed.

A mother who exclusively breast-feeds for the first 6 months may succeed in prolonging her periods to a certain extent.

But once a mother starts menstruating, she is like any other normal woman.

My advice to all couples would be to always be on the safer side and use a suitable method of contraception and space their children.

The advantages are:

1) The earlier child is well-fed on the breast and weaned properly as the mother can look after the child well.

2) Children spaced 3 years or more apart are born healthier.

3) The mother recovers her health. She can breast-feed her child in peace, eat well and replace the blood she lost during labour. She thus becomes mentally and physically fit to undergo another pregnancy.

There are several methods used for child spacing

a) **WITHDRAWAL METHOD:** Coitus or intercourse is interrupted by withdrawal of the penis just before ejaculation. The failure rate is high i.e., there are more chances of becoming pregnant and hence, an unsafe method.

b) **RHYTHM METHOD:** This is another natural method of child spacing. It can be applicable only in cases where ovulation, hence menstruation, occurs.

If a cycle of 28 days is considered, ovulation takes place 14 days before the first day of the periods. It is safe to have sex up to 7 days after the periods and 5 days just before the periods. The days prior to and after ovulation are unsafe, and sex on those days may cause conception. This method is known as the safe period and is relatively safer than withdrawal. It is applicable in those who menstruate at fixed intervals. For those with irregular or long-short intervals between menses, special calculations are required to find out their safe period, and they should consult their respective doctors.

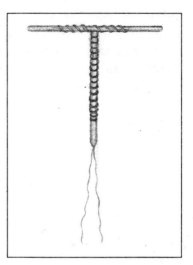

1●2●3●4●5 6 7 8 9 10 11 12 13 14 15 16 17 18 19 20 21 22 23 24 25 26 27 28
Ovulation

■ Safe Period

● Menses

Fig. 12.1, Diagrammatic representation of safe period in a 28 day cycle

c) CONDOMS: This is a barrier method, i.e. it creates a barrier between the cervix and discharging sperms. Condoms are also a relatively safer method. You need a cooperative male partner.

d) SPERMICIDAL SPONGES: These are small dissolving sponges containing chemicals which destroy sperms, hence preventing contraception. These sponges are to be placed in the cervix just before coitus. Properly used, these are also relatively safe. A popular brand TODAY is easily available.

e) ORAL CONTRACEPTIVE PILLS: Hormonal pills (Ovral, Mala-D, Mala-N, Triquilar, etc.) and non-hormonal pills (Saheli, Centron) are available.

Both types of pills are **absolutely contraindicated in lactating women.**

Fig. 12.2 : Copper-T

45

f) **INJECTABLE CONTRACEPTIVES:** Injections (Depo-provera) are also available and need to be taken once every three months. They do not have as many side-effects. They are also minimally secreted in the breast milk. These injections are one of the better methods of contraception for a lactating mother.

g) **I.U.C.D.:** Intra-uterine contraceptive devices are ones which, when placed in the uterus, prevent conception. The copper-T is such a device. It is inserted into the uterus about 6 weeks after the delivery, i.e., when the uterus returns to its normal size and position. This method is good for lactating mothers and even otherwise for child spacing.

How to Choose the Most Suitable Method.

Contraception and child spacing is like a pact between spouses. Depending upon the understanding between husband and wife and an open mind regarding family planning, any of the above methods can be used.

Condoms and the rhythm method are suitable for a compatible couple which does not want to use the hormonal injection or I.U.C.D.

For a woman who has the responsibility to prevent a new pregnancy all on herself, she could use the spermicidal sponge(TODAY), take the progesterone injection or insert an I.U.C.D

Isn't it a pity that there is no effective male contraceptive?

13

Breast-Feeding Under Special Condition

You have a Pair of Twins. How will You Feed Them?

Your body has prepared itself for the birth of twins, even if you do not know yourself.

Remember that more suckling makes more milk.

You can feed the twins together or one after the other.

Put a cushion on your lap, place the twins on the cushion and offer one breast each to the twins.

Sometimes each of them will feed on his or her favourite side.

If one twin is weaker than the other, make sure that the weaker one gets enough milk.

Of course, you will need the love and support of your near and dear ones. Difficulties will arise only because you have to look after two babies at the same time—and that is hard work.

Don't worry about your milk being less. Have the confidence to feed.

I know a mother with identical twins . She breast-fed them both. There were times when she got tired. But she was determined to feed them. She also had a good milk flow.
But her greatest advantage was that she was confident in her ability to produce milk:

Family History of Allergy

Allergies can be passed on from both parents to the child. Feeding on human milk is one of the best ways of reducing the risk of allergies.

Breast-milk, being genetically compatible with the infant, never causes allergic reactions. At the same time, due to its various contents, it induces anti-allergic resistance. If there is a family history of allergy, breast-feeding should be continued for as long as 2 years. At the same time, supplements given should not contain items known to cause allergy in the family. These items should be introduced slowly in the diet.

A normal infant's intestines are not mature enough to produce the disease and allergy-fighting proteins till the age 6 weeks. In an infant with a family history of allergy, these proteins are not produced till the age of 3 months. These are readily available in colostrum and breast milk.

Introducing cow's milk is a surefire way of inviting allergies as cow's milk protein is the commonest allergen. Cow's milk protein can cause skin reactions, cold (rhinitis), ear infection, respiratory infection, diarrhoea, poor weight gain, etc. Even introduction of formula foods at such an early age causes intolerance.

The infant outgrows intolerance to cow's milk by the age of 12 months and rarely shows any allergic reaction to cow's milk thereafter. Breast-milk only reduces the incidence of allergic reactions, and does not eliminate them.

Immunisation

Feeding after an injection of BCG, oral polio or triple vaccine does not cause any problems. You may feed the child afterwards if it is hungry.

What will you do if You get Pregnant while still Feeding Your Earlier Baby?

Most importantly, a pregnancy while feeding the

previous child should be absolutely avoided. With so many methods of prophylaxis very easily available in India, this should not be difficult.

If pregnancy is carried then breast-feeding of the earlier child needn't be stopped. There is no dilution or danger in feeding. Only when the milk physiologically turns back to colostrum in preparation of the new child, the earlier infant may be weaned or severed from the breast.

The danger here is malnutrition of the elder infant as it is not physiologically and mentally ready to be severed from the breast.

Continuing feeding even in the last trimester may sometimes cause uterine pain. Also, you can feed the elder and the new infant at the same time on your new milk-it is your wish entirely.

Mentally Handicapped Infant

Brain damage or retardation makes slow learners of the infants. Hence, they are poor feeders at the breast. Be patient and persevere. Never feel guilty. Your milk will keep the infant healthy and the mother-child bond will be maintained.

Low Birth Weight Infants

A low-birth weight infant (LBW) is one who, after a normal period of gestation, has lower weight than average, i.e., it is small for date.

A premature infant is one which is born before its expected date of delivery. These are invariably low-birth weight.

You Play an Important Role in the Care....

LBW infants have high protein requirement. They also need iron, calcium, vitamins and energy to grow.

Only your milk can provide all the necessary requirements. Plus breast-milk has the added advantages of being anti-allergic and anti-infective. Supplying your milk also helps you create your sense of attachment to the baby

Some of these LBW babies have difficulty in suckling.

Such babies should be given expressed milk. Express your milk as many times as you can, i.e., about 8-10 times in 24 hours and express as much milk as you can.

Don't leave long intervals between expressions. Feed the milk by cup or tube. DON'T USE A BOTTLE.

Feeds are approximately measured thus:

On the first day

60 ml of milk / kg baby's body weight.

Divide the total into 8 feeds. Feed every 3 hours

From the 2nd to the 7th day

Increase milk by 20 ml per day per kilo body weight, i.e., on the 2nd day give 80 ml /kg body weight.

On the 3rd day give 100 ml / kg body weight and so on.

From the 8th day

200 ml / kg body weight.

Continue feeding by cup till the baby can suckle. Weight should be regularly monitored on the growth chart.

Helping mothers to breast-feed. Indian adaptation by R.K. Anand.

Remember, there isn't any need to feel tense or stressed out. Only you can help your low-birth-weight baby.

Keep the baby warm and breast-feed well as your milk is the nectar that the baby needs to grow well and gain normal weight .

Don't ever try to give top feeds or water to the baby.

Donated expressed milk can also be given. STICK TO BREAST-MILK ONLY.

Don't get depressed. You are not helping the baby or yourself in any way. Breast-feed confidently.

You must continue exclusive breast-feeding after the baby is brought home.

Don't ever give top feeds or formulas.

You will run the risk of causing allergies and infections in the baby.

The feeds will also overload the delicate infant kidneys which is dangerous.

Also understand that an LBW baby does not have well developed intestines, so such food as cow's milk / formulas cannot be tolerated.

You must avoid bottle-feeding.

A point to note is that LBW infants are generally born to anaemic, undernourished mothers. So, a pregnant mother should be well nourished.

14

An Ill Infant

Mothers often wonder how they will be able to feed an ill baby. Here are some conditions and their solutions.

Obstruction to breathing

This could be:

1) CONGENITAL: At birth the baby has a structural defect like a cleft lip or palate. This causes problems in breathing while suckling. There could also be defects in the development of the nose. Such babies then refuse to suckle. Till surgical correction of these defects is done, expressed breast-milk should be fed either by spoon or *wati/katori* or by tube. The doctor will advise accordingly.

2) INFECTION: A common cold is the commonest cause of a blocked nose. The infant then uses its mouth to breathe. When held at the breast, the infant cannot breathe and starts fussing. The mother can try to clear the blocked nose with the help of a wisp of cotton. A small suction bulb is also available, which sucks out the mucous from the nose. Medication may be given after the doctor's advice.

Feeding should be resumed or the infant will get a fear of the breast thinking that it suffocates it.

Vomiting

Vomiting in an exclusively breast-fed baby gaining normal weight or passing urine normally does not need any treatment. If a baby is fussy, not putting on weight and is vomiting all feeds, then it needs to be examined by the doctor.

Overfed infants given formula feeds are the likeliest to regurgitate or vomit due to infection.

Once a baby is cured it should be breast-fed again.

Diarrhoea and Constipation

Exclusively breast-fed babies have two types of stool patterns.

1) Some infants pass loosely formed stools as many number of times as they are breast-fed. *This is not diarrhoea*. It is just that the child's intestines absorb what is required. The remaining excess and waste material is thrown out in stools.

   An exclusively breast-fed baby has minimal chances of getting infective diarrhoea as no other feeds, even water (whether boiled, filtered, etc.), is to be given for about 3-4 months. If such a child is not gaining weight, is not thriving and passes loose stools then there may be a problem.

   An infant who is on breast milk and also on other animal milks or fluids has a higher chance of getting infective diarrhoea.

2) Some infants do not pass stools at all for up to 5 days. These stools are infrequent but not hard. *This is not real constipation.* It is quite normal in exclusively breast-fed infants. If the mother is worried about the infant not passing stools, then every 2-3 days she can gently insert a wisp of cotton soaked in oil into the anal opening. The baby will pass stools. This procedure should not be made a habit.

The stool pattern of exclusively breast-fed babies varies from day to day. Someday they may pass as many as 10 stools and on somedays none. As long as the baby is thriving there is no cause for alarm.

Colic

This is said to occur because of increased bowel movements which cause discomfort. Most babies cry at a specific time every day. They are difficult to pacify. You may think the baby is hungry and put it to the breast, but this does not help.

Give slight pressure on the abdomen to relieve any "wind". Carminatives or antispasmodics may help. Consult a doctor before administering them.

Breast-feeding should be continued as normal. Colic disappears on its own.

Jaundice

There is an entity called *physiological jaundice* which occurs in most babies during the first fortnight after birth. This condition does not require any specific treatment as it starts, deepens and lessens on its own.

The child is active and suckles normally. It should be breast-fed as normal. Some babies become more sleepy and don't suckle properly. Give them expressed breast-milk by *wati/katori* or spoon every 3 hours.

Jaundice appearing within 24 hours after birth or in a child who appears unwell could be a cause for concern.

Fever

Any baby with fever is reluctant to suckle. Yet ,it needs its regular nutrition and extra fluids. Once the temperature is down the baby will start suckling. In the meanwhile, expressed breast-milk may be given by spoon and *wati/katori*. When the fever shoots up again the baby will refuse to suckle. A doctor's advice should be taken if a baby has fever.

Hospitalised Baby

Staying in a hospital for any illness is a traumatic experience for the infant as well as the mother. As a rule, mothers are allowed to stay with the child so that she can breast-feed her baby.

15

Normal Growth Of Baby

The anxiety over the normal growth of her infant is common to every mother.

Weighing the baby on a monthly basis and recording the weight on the chart helps to gauge growth. The chart is prepared such that the mother will know that her baby's weight is falling below average--implying malnutrition, or is higher than necessary--implying infantile obesity.

A normal baby weighs around 3 kgs at birth. The weight doubles by the fifth month and on the first birthday is about three times the birth weight.

A minute variation on the lower side must not be immediately considered as being due to inadequate breast-milk. Many mothers reach the conclusion that they just cannot produce more milk and rush to start formula feeds. There is no need for such a hurry.

Think. Is the home ambience conducive to you and your baby?

Is there anxiety during the process of feeding?

Are there relatives around who repeatedly say that your milk is not enough?

Has the baby failed to gain weight over a period of time? Is it just a one-time occurrence?

Is the positioning correct? Is your diet proper?

[5.1] Growth Chart

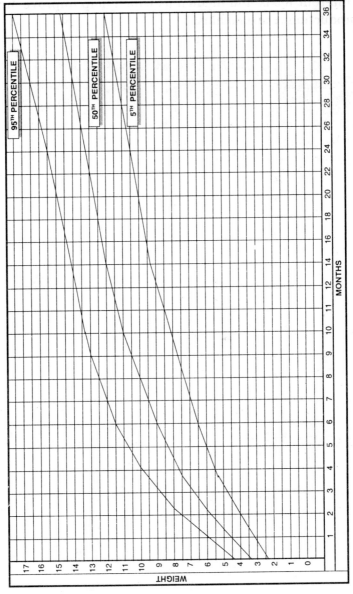

Fig. 15.1: Growth Chart

57

Patience, analysis of what could be wrong and determination will help. Galactogogues maybe tried. Different foods and medicines which help improve milk production cause no harm.

16

Can You Breast-Feed If You Suffer From...?

Common Cold and Cough

Viruses cause common cold and cough which affect every person. It is a self limiting condition, i.e. goes, away with or without treatment. Don't worry about your child being infected because the child is anyway exposed to all micro-organisms harboured by the you. *Continue breast-feeding*. Consult a doctor if you need medicines.

Tuberculosis

Anyone can be infected by TB. If a mother is suffering from TB then she has to take a 6-9 months course like every infected person. This is not a contraindication for breast-feeding. Initially thought of as dangerous, *breastmilk can be breast-fed to the child* even if its mother has got TB.

In an open case of TB, the mother should express her milk and feed by spoon or *wati.*

Once her state of infection reduces (the doctor will tell when) she can put the child to her breast. This way she ensures continuous production of breast milk and her child gets breast milk from day one.

Leprosy

A mother can breast-feed her baby.

Cancer

Pregnancy itself is not advisable for a woman having cancer.unlike the movies. But if a woman is unfortunate enough to have been diagnosed as suffering after her delivery, she *should not breast-feed at all*. This is because the treatment could harm the infant's growth and development.

AIDS

HIV positive cases are more common than full blown AIDS. Testing for HIV is mandatory for all pregnant women. The child is also tested for HIV after birth. *If the mother and child both are HIV positive, then breast-feeding can be done*. At least the breast milk will provide nutrition. *If* the *mother* is HIV *positive* and the *child is* HIV *negative* then she has the following options:

1) Use the services of a wet nurse to feed her baby.
2) She can express her milk, pasteurise it and feed the baby. Pasteurisation is the treatment of milk by heating it to 56°C for 30 minutes followed by rapid cooling to 12°C on ice *(Training manual on breast-feeding management. Steps towards baby friendly care by UNICEF)*.
3) Donated, expressed breast milk (EBM) can be fed.
4) A mother's own expressed milk but boiled. Boiling breast milk though. destroys certain protective factors.

If an HIV positive mother can avail of a wet nurse or donated EBM then she must use them. If not, she should preferably use her own expressed pasteurised milk. Boiled breast milk should be the last option.

Jaundice

There are different types of infective hepatitis. I shall talk about some commonly seen viral hepatitis.

If a lactating mother has HEPATITIS A, she can *continue feeding.*

A mother with HEPATITIS B infection *can also breast-feed* her baby provided the child is immunized against Hepatitis B. There is no increased risk.

HEPATITIS C (HCV) maybe transmitted through breast milk. Hence, a mother thus infected should *look into other alternatives* like a wet nurse or donated EBM.

Malaria

A mother can continue breast-feeding.

Caesarean Section

It should not be considered an illness. Lactation is initiated, depending upon the mother's post-operative condition. If regional anaesthesia has been given, then the mother is conscious as in a normal delivery. The baby can be put to the breast within an hour. If the mother has been given general anaesthesia, as soon as she recovers from the effects of anaesthesia, she should put the baby to her breast. *There is no connection between a caesarean and so-called low production or absence of breast milk.* These myths are perpetuated by people surrounding the mother.

Sit, relax, use cushions, whatever is comfortable and painless. If the mother is lying down and finds it difficult to get up, yet wants to feed her baby, she can do so by shifting her position. As long as the nipple and breast are within the baby's reach it will suckle. Expressed colostrum and breast milk can also be given.

YOU CAN RESTART YOUR MILK PRODUCTION!

There are times when breast-feeding may be reduced or stopped. You may feel that the milk will dry up and so there is no point in continuing breast-feeding. This is a fallacy. Milk production can be increased. *Determination and confidence are the keys.*

You know that the stimulation for production and let down are suckling. Put to the infant to the breast for short and frequent duration—about 5 minutes, 10 to 15 times a day.

Within 10-15 days a confident mother will be relactating. Anxiety and doubt will lengthen the time for relactation, which will in turn increase stress. You may feel it is nonsense. *Don't stop bothering or trying.* NEVER give top feeds before putting it to the breast. On a full stomach the infant will not suckle and the stimulus will fail. Top feeds can be given by spoon or *wati* after the baby has suckled and taken in the milk produced. Gradually the milk will increase and the supplements can be reduced. Why a new mother, even a non-pregnant woman can fully or partially be able to feed a child. The only stimulus is a sucking child. It will take time, of course, but it can be done. It has happened.

One should try.

17

Expressing And Storing Milk

Expression of milk
Expression or removal of breast-milk can be done by the methods mentioned below. This is a necessary procedure for those mothers who want to maintain the continuity of breast-feeding but cannot actually breast-feed due to various reasons.

Manual Expression (by hand)
This is a simple way of expressing milk. The only precaution needed is washing of hands. This prevents contamination of the milk by the micro-organisms present in the skin and nails.

One breast at a time is taken.

★ Wash and clean both hands thoroughly.

★ Gently massage the breasts.

★ Put the thumb above the nipple and the forefinger below the nipple on the areola.

★ Press both towards the chest wall.

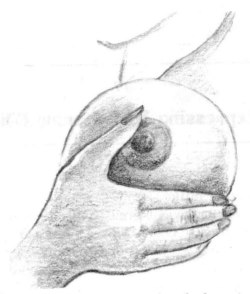

Fig. 17.1 : Gently massaging the breast

★ Gently squeeze the areola behind the nipple, betwee the thumb and forefinger.

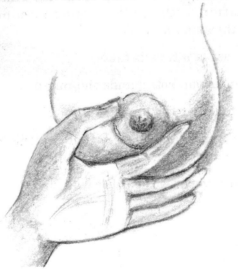

Fig. 17.2 : Squeezing the areola : rest of the fingers supporting the breast

★ Continue the action of squeezing and releasing.
★ The areola can be pressed from above and below and from the sides of the nipple as well.
★ Express from one breast. When the milk flow reduces, change to the other breast and express in a similar fashion.
★ Collect the milk in a wide-mouthed cup or glass which has been washed and cleaned with hot water and soap.
   If the process is painful-then you are not doing it correctly.

Always be in a comfortable position while expressing milk.

Breast Pump

These are of two types:

a) MANUAL BREAST PUMP: The one type most commonly available is shaped like a trumpet. There is a funnel-shaped plastic, the end of which is fixed into a rubber bulb. A round protrusion of the plastic is present towards the end of the funnel for collection of milk.

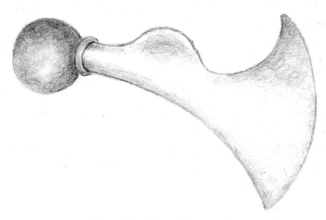

Fig. 17.3 : Breast pump

The funnel is placed on the breast in such a way that the nipple and areola lie at the centre. The edges of the funnel are firmly in contact with the breast skin, to prevent any air entry. The rubber bulb is pressed to create suction and then released. The bulb springs back to its original shape, creating negative pressure. The nipple is pulled into the stem of the funnel. Repeating the action induces the ejection reflex and milk flows. It collects in the small protrusion towards the end of the funnel. The collected milk is then either fed or stored. Sterilise the pump before each use.

In foreign countries a variety of breast pumps are available. These can be easily obtained.

b) ELECTRIC BREAST PUMP: This is commonly used in hospitals to collect milk.

Manual expression is to be preferred to use of any type of breast pump.

Storage of Milk

Collect the milk in a wide-mouthed cup or glass. Wash it with hot water and soap before collecting the milk.

It stays good at room temperature for 8 hours.

One can also keep the covered container inside the refrigerator (not in the door) for 24 hours. It can be warmed by placing the container in a bowl of warm water.

There isn't any need to boil the milk as it loses its anti-infective properties. It should be used raw.

This milk can thus be utilised in one working day. Feed by cup or spoon. Don't use the bottle.

Before feeding, shake the container to remix the floating fat globules with the rest of the milk.

18

Breast-Feeding And Medications

The drugs you take are secreted in your milk.

These Drugs to be Completely Avoided

*anti-cancer   *anti-thyroid   *radioactive preparations
*lead   *mercury   *lithium   *immune suppressants
*gold   *morphine   *ergot (a single dose may be given but just that)

Drugs having Mild Side effects

*oral contraceptives   *tetracyclines   *chloramphenicol
*nitrofurantoin   *metronidazole   *sulphonamides
*sulphonylureas   *aspirin   *indomethacin
*magnesium sulphate

Drugs that can be taken without Causing Harm to the Baby

*non-narcotic pain killers   *anti-hypertensives   *anti-asthma   *antibiotics (other than tetracycline, sulphonamides and chloramphenicol) *tranquilisers *isabgol) (other laxatives are contraindicated)

THIS LIST DOES NOT IMPLY THAT THE DRUGS ARE COMPLETELY HARMLESS.

Galactogogues

Like foods which help to improve milk production, there are some drugs which help increase milk production.

Allopathic drugs are:
Metaclopramide and synthetic oxytocin.

Ayurvedic drugs are indigenous to India and have been used for centuries. They are:
*shatavari *kakoli *jeevanti *kamboji.

> **ALL DRUGS SHOULD BE TAKEN AFTER CONSULTING A DOCTOR WHO IS WELL INFORMED ABOUT THE SUBJECT OF BREAST-FEEDING AND MEDICATIONS.**

Inhibition of Milk Secretion

Some mothers unfortunately may give birth to a still born child or the infant may die due to an illness or a congenital deformity. In such cases, the mothers body continues to form breast milk for sometime at least.

There are two choices she can make:

a) She can offer to feed the infant of a mother whose milk production is low and hence not enough for her baby.

b) She can stop her milk production with the help of medication.

BROMOERGOCRYPTINE: This drug helps in suppressing milk production. It should be taken under medical supervision only.

You can also tightly bind your breasts and take a painkiller to reduce the pain. In the absence a of stimulus, milk production will automatically reduce and stop.

19

You Are A Working Woman...

So, you know most of what is to be known about breast-feeding.

But, how does that solve your problem? You work and still want to feed.

First of all you should remember that breast-feeding is a basic right—yours and that of your child.

Secondly, you must not feel guilty about working. You work because you want a career or for economic reasons. Neither is a crime.

Most Indian companies offer up to 3 months paid maternity leave to all pregnant employees. Some offer up to 6 months paid leave and some the option of extending the leave up to 6 months. Various private companies offer flexitime work for their female employees so that they may work from office and home and look after the baby.

The International Labour Organisation (ILO) and the United Nations (UN) have recognised this need of working women and have recommended legislative changes to all countries.

India, China and other East Asian countries, the Arab world and some European countries are among those who have adopted these changes.

Your employers are not doing you a favour by granting you leave.

Take the entire 3 months leave and if possible, extend it to 6 months. You can start your child on supplements by then. But, breast milk still needs to be given.

Trying to Maintain Milk after Returning to Work

Feeding at the same frequency as the earlier months is difficult. If you are determined you can do it.

To maintain the milk the main stimulus is suckling.

For that you have some options:

1) Some employers offer creche facilities within the office premises or nearby, allowing you to feed the baby at intervals. You must take advantage of it.
   But, I don't see many mothers carrying their infants from farflung suburbs to the office on crowded buses and trains.

2) Express and store your milk so that it can be fed to the baby (by spoon, *wati / katori*, a small glass, a cup or a *bondla*) when you go for work. As you know, your milk, if properly stored, stays unspoilt for 8 hours at room temperature.

3) Feed your child during the day before leaving for work, in the evening when you get back and during the night.

4) Breast-feed more during holidays.

You must add supplements by the age of 5-6 months.

This way, working women will not have problems for as long as they want to feed.

20

Irrational Practices In Breast-Feeding

There are some ridiculous practices prevalent in our society which are really detrimental to the act of breast-feeding.

They are:

a) The infant being whisked away after delivery to the sterile nursery. The hospital staff have decided that you are too tired to hold or feed your baby. Your baby is physically bound to you and needs your warmth and closeness for security. The few days you spend in the hospital are for learning to handle your baby with the help of skilled hospital staff. You are not meant to see your infant like a rare piece of art brought out at feeding times (which, by the way, are decided by the staff).

b) Discarding colostrum. You have read about the importance of colostrum earlier, so you know why it can't be discarded.

c) A method in which the infant is before and after every feed, just to check on the rate of growth is called *test weighing*. Breast milk varies from feed to feed in amount. The infant too does not always have the same amount at every feed. Test weighing gives inconsistent results. There is a high margin of error in the measurements. Most importantly, the mother's level of stress increases, affecting milk production and let down. A check on the weight is necessary only if the mother is a low producer or has irregular ejection. Then also test weighing is not advisable. Weight can be taken every 3-4 days. Remember, there is physiological weight loss in the first week after birth which is regained in 10-15 days.

d) Feeding glucose to the infant as its first feed. There is no rationale behind this action. This is continued till the mother secretes milk. Instead, infection may be introduced due to the water.

e) Deciding edibility according to the colour of the milk.

f) Collecting some milk and putting a fly in it to decide the fat content.

g) Feeding by the clock, i.e, every hour or 2 hours. How can the hospital staff or anyone decide the exact time for a feed? The best person to know is the infant.

h) Feeding for fixed times is also wrong. Again, the infant decides for how long it wants to suckle.

i) You will be advised to give only one breast at a time or feed at one breast only all the time. Breasts can be changed during a feed.

The point to remember here is that you must not withdraw a breast suddenly mid-feed. If you do that, the baby will have got only foremilk and not hindmilk. As you know by now, hindmilk, having a higher fat content, is more filling and supplies more energy. So, if due to a breast change mid-feed, the infant does not get hindmilk, it will remain hungry. The best way to ensure uniform emptying and shape maintenance is to offer alternate breasts after every feed.

21

Mother-Child Bond—One Of Its Kind

The birth of your child induces overwhelming, indescribable emotions within you. The immediate feeling is that of giving care to the infant. This is natural. In the womb the baby can hear your heart-beat and feel your warmth. After birth, skin-to skin contact, hearing your heart-beat when held close to the body, your body warmth, recognising your voice will reassure the infant of its position in the new world. It develops a sense of security. The act of breast-feeding only enhances these feelings. There is eye to eye contact of the mother and child, a communication beyond words. Removal of the infant immediately after birth to a sterile, clean nursery deprives the infant of all this. Lack of body warmth, skin to skin contact, hearing the mother's voice, heart beat, etc. deprive the infant of its initial emotional security. The natural maternal caring skills that a mother feels immediately post-delivery are lost. Carrying the infant on the back is seen as an extension of the initial mother-child contact.The infant is not disturbed by the movements of the mother, it has been used to them since the foetal stage. In the hurly-burly of daily life, the importance of the mother child-bond has been overlooked or considered insignificant by some. Following maternal instinct and wanting close contact with the infant never causes harm to the mother or child.

Sudden Weaning

There are instances when a mother, who is breast-feeding her child, is pregnant with the second. Birth of the second child means sudden cessation of breast-feeding for the first in most cases. Can you imagine the plight of such a child? The mother has no time for the child. She is busy looking after her new baby, which is time-consuming. The elder child is left to its own devices. Deprived of maternal warmth, the child indulges in attention-attracting activities. It throws tantrums and cries, for which it is punished. It is but natural for such a child to be miserable and insecure.

Such a mother has two options:

1) To prevent a pregnancy for at least 2 years after the birth of the first child.

2) If there is a pregnancy, gradually wean the child over a period of 2-3 months. Continue breast feeding of the elder child along with the newborn. It causes no harm.

Psychological Advantage of Breast-feeding over Bottle-feeding

Picture two infants, one with its mother breast-feeding and the other being fed by a bottle.

The bottle-fed infant is lying by itself holding the bottle, or someone holding it . There is no eye to eye contact, no warmth. Skin to skin contact is missing and the opportunity for bonding with the mother is decreased, sometimes completely absent.

In total contrast, the breast-fed infant is ensconced in the mother's arms. It can hear her heart beats, smell her closeness, play with her breast, be cuddled. This contact is not only reassuring to the child but pleasurable to the mother and ensures maintenance of lactation.

Think of the sense of security that each breast-fed child will have. Doesn't that make-breast-feeding superior to the bottle?

74

22

Supplementation And Weaning

What is Supplementation?
The word supplement means "to add".
An infant is given supplements because:
1) insufficient breast milk is secreted by the mother, causing failure to increase body weight —which may happen in the early months of life.
2) the physiological demands grow with age and breast milk alone cannot provide the body's needs.

What is Weaning?
The term weaning is commonly though wrongly used to imply stoppage of breast-feeding.

"To wean" actually means to accustom to other foods.

Introducing Supplementary Feeds
Mothers with proven low milk will need to introduce supplements earlier.

Considering that a mother has adequate breast-milk, supplementary feeds can be introduced at about 6 months of age.

Supplementary feeds do not imply only other animal milks fed by bottle. They include other liquids, porridges, soups, mashed fruits and other animal milks fed by spoon or *wati / katori*. Supplements also do not mean marketed formula foods.

For the period prior to introduction of supplementary feeds, the baby should be exclusively breast-fed. There is no need to give water also as human milk contains a good amount of water.

Starting supplementary feeds does not mean that the nutritional efficacy of breast-milk has reduced. Only the demands of the body have increased. The quality of milk is excellent and it still forms an important part of a child's diet.

Introduce the feeds in small amounts and give in place of a breast-feed or after a feed. The quantity of the feed should be small and the frequency often. This can be given over a period of several months with breast milk up to 1½-2 years.

What is the Ideal Duration of Breast-feeding?

Those who do not advocate breast-milk at all, say there is no need to start breast-feeding anyway.

Then there are those who feed forever and ever, i.e., up to age of 5 and sometimes above. The tendency in these cases is to hold the child to the breast whenever it cries. Instead of trying to find the reason as to why it is crying, the mother prefers to put it to the breast and keep the child quiet. Think of the psychological effect such prolonged feeding can have on the child.

Some mothers believe that the longer they breast-feed, the longer they can avoid pregnancy. (This is a very common but obviously wrong belief.)

This is physiologically impossible.

THE IDEAL DURATION OF BREAST FEEDING ALONG WITH SUPPLEMENTATION IS 1½-2 YEARS.

By this age the child has developed its milk teeth and can chew adult food.

Most children begin to lose interest in breast milk when fed adult foods and stop demanding it.

A mother should never have to stop breast-feeding because everyone has told her to. Decide after considering the ideal period and accordingly start supplements and weaning.

How to Wean

Introduction of supplementary foods not only fulfil the growing body demands of the child, but also act as weaning foods.

The child gets accustomed to tastes other than breast milk.

This is very important. Sevrage or sudden cessation leaves the child hungry and frustrated. It has not yet developed a taste for other foods and cannot get breast milk because the mother feels it is high time it started on other foods. This leads to undernutrition.

"Development of taste" is very important if you do not want to have a fussy child who refuses to eat well in its growing years (a common complaint from age 2-3 years).

Weaning can be done in steps as follows:

At 6 months to 9 months

Start with fruits like mashed ripe banana, thin rava kheer, fruit juices, mashed vegetables like potatoes, carrots, soups, coconut water, seasonal fruits, apple pulp, papaya, etc.e.g. Take a quarter overripe banana to begin with. Increase by a quarter every week till the limit accepted. Banana can be interchanged with other fruits.

Then introduce various porridges, home-made weaning mixes (see below), moong, tur dal, mashed green leafy vegetables.

At about 8 months add egg and other soft meats.

At 9 months to 12 months

Soft cooked rice, plain dal and other foods eaten by the family. Only it should be less spicy and soft in consistency.

Fruits, vegetables, dahi, buttermilk, etc., should be given in the earlier months.

Breast-feeding should be continued.

By 12 months the child should be sharing the family meal, albeit in smaller quantities.

★ Start with one food item at a time, enabling the baby to get used to it.

★ Give semi-solids initially and gradually shift to solids over 2-3 weeks. These supply more energy.

★ Adding oil/ghee, sugar/ jaggery to the home-made mixes increases the energy density, keeping the volume of the feed small.

★ Remember, breast-feed first and then give the other feed. Or, give the feed between breast-feeds. As the food intake increases, the intervals between breast-feeds also increases.

★ Families with history of allergy should introduce foods like egg cocoa, artificial milk, and these should never be given to an infant in the first 6 months of life.

A suggested schedule for giving these feeds is:

2-4 times a day at 6-8 months.

4-6 times a day at 9-12 months.

(Training manual on breast-feeding management. Steps towards baby friendly care by UNICEF).

It is essential that you learn to balance between these foods and breast-milk. All children will invariably show distaste towards other foods. That does not mean you should give up these foods and go back to your old routine.

Understand that your baby is growing and requires to be put on weaning foods along with breast-milk.

Home-made Mixes

Why is it that mothers, once they start supplementation and weaning, buy marketed foods?

Most would say that they are easy to prepare, convenient to carry, have the necessary ingredients and the whole world uses them, so why not me?

Apart from being expensive, marketed foods can lead to allergies and diarrhoeas.

Home-made mixes have been used before the advent of marketed foods, are simple to prepare, and the contents are known.

There are minimal chances of allergies, diarrhoeas, and other conditions.

The cost of home-made mixes do not burn a hole in the pocket.

The **National Institute of Nutrition** has prepared recipes for home-made supplements. These are low-cost foods, prepared from locally available foodstuffs, easy to cook and of acceptable taste, bulk, colour and consistency. *These supplements are meant for infants of about 6 months of age.*

Table 22.1 : Wheatgram Porridge

Ingredients	Amount
1) Roasted wheat flour	25 grams (1½ tablespoons)
2) Powdered roasted bengalgram	15 grams (1 tablespoon)
3) Powdered roasted groundnut	10 grams (2 teaspoons)
4) Jaggery/ sugar	30 grams (2 tablespoons)
5) Spinach/ any other green leafy vegetable	30 grams

a) Mix the wheat flour, bengal gram and groundnut powders.

b) Dissolve the jaggery/ sugar in a small amount of water to form a syrup.

c) Prepare a batter of the syrup and flour+powder mixture.

d) Boil the spinach/ green leafy vegetable in water till soft. Mash and strain through a clean cloth to prepare the vegetable soup.

e) Add the vegetable soup to the batter and cook with continuous stirring till semi-solid.

The flour + powder mixture can be mixed in larger amounts and stored in the refrigerator.

Table 22.2 : Rice Porridge

	Ingredients		Amount
1)	Rice	30 grams	(2 tablespoons)
2)	Powdered roasted groundnut	15 grams	(1 tablespoon)
3)	Powdered roasted greengram/ redgram dal	10 grams	(3/4 tablespoon)
4)	Jaggery/sugar	30 grams	(2 tablespoons)
5)	Spinach/ green leafy vegetable	30 grams	

a) Cook the rice.
b) Add the dal and groundnut powder to the cooked rice and mix.
c) Prepare a soup of the green leafy vegetable by boiling in water till soft. Mash and strain through a clean cloth for the soup.
d) Add the jaggery/ sugar to the above mixture.
e) Cook for a few minutes.

Table 22.3 : Ragi (Millet) Infant Food

Ingredients		Amount
1) Dehusked and roasted ragi	45 grams	(3 tablespoons)
2) Roasted green gram dal	20 grams	(1¼ tablespoon)
3) Roasted groundnut	10 grams	(¾ tablespoon)
4) Roasted decorticated til	5 grams	(1 teaspoon)
5) Jaggery/ sugar	30 grams	(2 tablespoons)

a) Soak the ragi in water overnight. Drain the water, spread the grains on a plate and allow to germinate by covering with a damp cloth for one day. Dry the germinated ragi in the sun, roast till it develops a malted flavour. Then powder it.

b) Powder the other ingredients individually. Mix with ragi powder and store in an airtight container.

c) Take suitable amounts from the mixture (60-70 grams or 4 tablespoons) and mix with a small amount of water or milk to make a paste for feeding.

Make sure to use only healthy looking groundnuts. Shrivelled, fungus-covered nuts may lead to problems on consumption.

Table 22.4 : Rice Khichdi

Ingredients	Amount
1) Cooked rice	1 cup
2) Cooked pulse(red/ green gram)	1/2 cup
3) Cooked leafy vegetable	2 tablespoons
4) Jaggery/ sugar	3 teaspoons
5) Oil	1 teaspoon

a) Mix the cooked rice and cooked pulse.

b) Mash the cooked leafy vegetable with additional water and strain through a clean cloth to prepare the soup.

c) Add the soup and the required seasonings to the above mixture.

d) Add the sugar/ jaggery and mix well.

Danger Period

The period since the initiation of weaning till complete stoppage of breast milk is very crucial.

This is generally 6 months to 2 years. Growth is fastest then.

Lack of optimal nutrients may have long-term effects on the growth potential and health of these children.

Do not try to inculcate adult habits such as meals at fixed times and only twice or three times a day. This habit can be formed when the child is able to sit with the rest of the family at meal times. Otherwise the child should be fed whenever hungry. Either milk or a mix.

Market Feeds

The benefits of formula or market feeds are reaped by the parent company and never by the consumer.

Except in very rare cases where premixed instant food is needed, home-made mixes will do.

Breast-feeding can never be replaced by these foods. While purchasing, which should preferably be avoided, take care to check the contents and method of preparation. Many times a small though vital ingredient is missing and may continue to be deficient, leading to unwanted disease conditions.

23

Dangers Of Bottle-Feeding And Early Weaning

Bottle-feeding means feeding cow's milk or prepared dried milk powders or formula feeds in place of breast milk.

It is fashionable but has a lot of disadvantages.

a) Bottle feeding makes the infant exercise more mouth muscles for sucking than it would with the breast. This tires the baby. A lot of air is also taken in while bottle feeding, which gives a sense of fullness to the stomach.

b) The time factor is also to be considered. Sterilising the bottle and teat before every feed, preparing the mixture after measuring the correct amounts of milk or powder and water are time consuming procedures.

c) It is two or three times more expensive to bottle-feed an infant with formulas than to provide a lactating mother the necessary extra nutrients from everyday less costly foods.

d) Iron deficiency anaemia is so common in Indian women that a child born to an anaemic woman also has deficient iron stores. Bottle-feeding such an infant only aggravates the anaemia. Cow's milk and human milk have the same iron content. The difference is that human milk also contains more vitamin C, copper and vitamin E which help the absorption of iron in the infant's intestines. Cow's milk contains these in less amount, and formula feeds probably none. A tendency to minute bleeding of the intestines is seen in bottle-fed infants. These bleedings lead to further loss of iron in the form of blood.

.e) Calcium deficiency is common in children fed on cow's milk. This is because the calcium present in cow's milk is poorly absorbed up by the infant's body. This deficiency of calcium in bottle-fed infants leads to convulsions and heart failure. Apart from these immediate risks, the enamel of the teeth is weakened, causing dental defects.

f) The sodium content of cow's milk is very high as compared to human milk. This leads to an overload on the infant's kidneys which the kidneys may not be able to bear and is very dangerous.

g) The thought that a plump baby is a healthy baby leads to competition between mothers who want their baby to be the best. Overfeeding in the form of dual feeds, i.e., bottle-feeding, and semi-solids in the earlier months itself, leads to a condition called infantile obesity. The mother coaxes her baby to take in more than required. This causes excess calorie intake. Few calories are used, making the infant fat and sluggish.

In contrast, breast milk intake depends upon the baby. So each time it feeds the right amount. Very few breast-fed babies have infantile obesity.

h) Cow's milk protein and the proteins in formula feeds are alien to the baby's body. This causes allergy or sensitivity as the infant's immunity has not yet developed. Early weaning by eggs, fruits, fish, etc., is also an invitation to allergies.

i) The anti-infective properties of breast milk have been explained. Breast-feeding protects against a multitude of infections. Chest infection, ear infection, diarrhoea and vomiting are more common in bottle-fed than in breast-fed infants.

A normal breast-fed baby's intestines harbour bacteria which are essential for the process of digestion. These "home grown", non-disease causing bacteria do not cause any infection and are in fact essential not only for digestion but also in the synthesis of vitamins B complex. In a bottle-fed baby, instead of such "normal" bacteria, the intestines favour the growth of disease-causing organisms which give rise to infective diarrhoea.

In my practice, I see several infants with chest infections, ear infections, skin disease, diarrhoea, etc.

Do you know what is common to all these babies?

They are all on the bottle and "dabba", started as early as the 1st or 2nd month of life.

A pity that some mothers don't know how their milk can make healthy babies.

j) As teeth develop, they are prone to decay. This is very peculiar in bottle-fed infants, who sleep with the bottle in the mouth and continue sucking. It happens because, instead of being completely swallowed, the milk stagnates around the gums. The excess sugar content in the formula or prepared milk is a breeding ground for bacteria. The absence of fluoride in the formula or cow's milk also causes dental caries.

k) The teeth do not develop properly. They are mostly protruding to various degrees and need to be corrected. The difference in the mechanism of sucking between breast-feeding and bottle-feeding is said to lead to this condition.

l) The curd formed by cow's milk is denser than that of breast milk. This curd is hard and rubbery, causing obstruction in the infant's intestines, which is serious.

Now you know!
Breast-milk is the best milk.
It is ready-to-use.
It is custom-made.
Available at room temperature.
Easy to feed.
And almost free!

Why Feed with a Small Glass, a *Katori (wati)*, a Bondla or a Spoon?

In case you cannot breast-feed or want to feed your expressed milk, an ordinary small glass or cup should be preferred to a bottle.

The dangers of bottle-feeding are not associated with the feeding cup.

Traditionally also, ancient cultures in India and other countries have been using horns or leaves like the banana flower leaf to feed artificially. The feeding cup is similar in shape to the banana flower leaf. In Marathi, the feeding cup is called *bondla*.

The feeding cup is easily available in stainless steel. If not, a spoon or *wati / katori* can be used. Of course, the precaution of cleanliness should be taken.

24

Composition Of Human Milk
Why It Is Most Suitable For Your Baby

"Breast is best". You must have heard this phrase so many times. Isn't it?

Wouldn't you like to know why ?

Don't think that only the "vernacular" or the "old fashioned" breast-feed. They do so only because it is the "done" thing. Most of them don't know why they are doing it.

I am going to tell you why you should breast-feed. For that you have to understand the contents of your milk .

Colostrum
This yellow viscous fluid is secreted prior to breast milk.

It is sometimes secreted from the third trimester of pregnancy itself.

It is an absolute necessity for every infant. Never discard it.

It is made up of:

FATS: These supply energy to the baby.

PROTEINS: They help in fighting diseases and build the resistance of your baby.

LACTOSE: This is a sugar which gives sweetness and helps in making more energy.

ZINC: This helps in preventing skin diseases.

SODIUM, POTASSIUM. CALCIUM, MAGNESIUM, PHOSPHORUS, etc., are also present

VITAMINS: Plenty of them are present in colostrum.

Like blood, colostrum contains *disease fighting cells* to a lesser extent.

> **Colostrum is highly nutritious.**
> **It is anti-allergic.**
> **It is anti-infective.**
> **It also helps in clearing the intestines of stools.**
> **Never discard it.**

Breast (Human) Milk

To look at, human milk is a thin fluid, white in colour with a tinge of blue.

It is made up of:

PROTEINS: Human milk contains various proteins having different functions.

They have anti-bacterial effects.

There are disease-fighting proteins which play a major role in the initial resistance build-up of the infant, till its own immune system starts functioning properly.

They play a vital role in the metabolism taking place in the body.

Your milk is the only source of non-allergic proteins for the infant.

Deficiency can lead to several disease conditions.

These proteins are divided into groups and sub-groups, all with specific functions which are all necessary for, normal growth of the baby.

Protein deficiency can lead to protein energy malnutrition which can be fatal.

FATS: The initial milk that comes out during a feed is called *foremilk*.

The last milk is called *hindmilk*. It has a higher fat content than foremilk.

The main functions of fat are to supply calories, vitamins and fatty acids essential to the body.

The human nervous system (the brain, nerves, etc) is made up of mostly fatty substances.

For the development of the infant's nervous system, fat is a requisite.

Essential fatty acids are present in human milk and needed by the nervous system for its build-up.

The human brain is what makes a human the most powerful mammal on earth.

It grows the fastest during infancy.

Energy is also available faster through breast-milk.

A baby needs foremilk and hindmilk for growth. Do not take a slow-feeding baby off the breast before it finishes. This will leave the baby dissatisfied and hungry as it hasn't got enough hindmilk

LACTOSE: This is a sugar. Only one sugar is found in breast-milk.

This is what gives milk its sweetness and taste.

It plays a major role in the development of the infant's nervous system, like fats.

It prevents calcium-deficiency conditions.

It prevents growth of disease-causing bacteria in the child's intestines.

IRON: The iron content of your milk is just right for the infant.

A normal newborn baby has its own iron stores in the liver which are used for preparing haemoglobin and the formation of red blood cells.

An overload of iron is harmful.

The iron in human milk helps in prevention of nutritional anaemia and is almost always adequate for the infant's needs.

SALTS AND WATER: Human milk is a thin watery fluid, i.e. it is rather dilute. The salts—sodium, potassium and chlorides--are low in content.

If they were high, the load on the baby's kidney would be too much.

The advantage of high water content is that extra water feeds are not required.

The body takes up whatever amount is needed and excretes the rest through urine.

Even in hot humid climates, exclusively breast-fed babies do not need extra water as the body gets what it needs through the human milk. Only ill infants need extra water.

CALCIUM: The calcium in breast-milk is completely utilised by the infant's body.

TRACE ELEMENTS: Zinc, copper, iodine, fluoride, manganese, cobalt, selenium, chromium, etc., are all trace elements and each one plays a role in the growth and maturity of the infant, and build-up of immunity, e.g., zinc helps in the prevention of skin diseases, generally seen in bottle-fed infants. Similarly, copper and zinc together help in the prevention of heart diseases.

Fluoride prevents dental caries and iodine helps in normal growth.

VITAMINS: The vitamins are present in plentiful in a mother who eats normal everyday food properly. There are "vitamin binders" in human milk. They are released in the infant's body. These vitamin binders are also said to have anti-bacterial activity after release of the vitamins.

CELLS: Just as human blood contains cells, so does human milk.

As you know, these cells are also present in colostrum.

Not only do they fight diseases but also produce substances which build immunity.

The Quran mentions human milk as "white blood", probably due to this very quality.

Why is Your Milk Most Suitable for Your baby?
All mammals secrete milk which suits only their babies.
So, camel milk is suitable only for a baby camel.

Even cow's milk is basically suitable for a calf.

Let us compare your milk with the cow's milk and you
will know why your milk is most suitable for your baby.

Contents	Human Milk	Cow's Milk
Proteins	Protein forms soft, flocculent curds in the intestines. Easy to digest.	Protein forms tough, rubbery curds. Difficult to digest. May cause intestinal obstruction.
Fats	Used for the development of the nervous system. Energy available faster.	Do not help in development of nervous system. Energy not available fast.
Sugar (lactose)	Enhances calcium absorption, is used in the development of the nervous system, prevents growth of disease-causing bacteria.	Does not help in calcium absorption or development of nervous system. Cow's milk fed infants may have disease causing bacteria in their intestines.
Iron	Is just right. Does not overload.	Drinking cow's milk causes minute bleeding in the intestines, leading to iron loss.
Salts & Water	The dilute nature of breast milk balances salts and water. Both are as needed by the body. Extra water feeds not needed. Hence, chances of waterborne disease is nil. increases.	More salts and less water increase load on kidney. Baby's thirst increases. Needs extra water to quench thirst. Hence risk of diarrhoea and other infections

Calcium	Utilisation is more	Utilisation is less leading to calcium deficiency.
Trace Elements	These trace elements are more useful for better growth than those of cow's milk.	Trace elements not well taken up by the baby's body.
Vitamins	Vitamins A and C are more. Concentration of other vitamins varies depending upon your baby's needs. Vitamin C helps in absorption of iron.	Vitamins A and C are less Others vary in amount as needed by a calf. Vitamins not so well utilised by your baby's body.

Now you know that your milk is unique. No market formula or animal milk can ever be a substitute.

25

Advantages Of Breast-Feeding

You now know a lot of things regarding breast milk and feeding. You also know the composition of your breast milk. Under this heading, I have put together all the advantages you will have if you breast-feed your baby.

Your Milk Protects against Infections...
Human milk contains several factors which have protective properties and /or trigger mechanisms within the body to fight infection.

As you know, human milk prevents growth of disease causing bacteria in the intestines which, in fact, protect against infections.

As is common knowledge, the human skin itself harbours micro-organisms and the breast skin is no exception. These organisms mix with the secreted milk. Yet, they never cause infections because of the anti-infective properties of human milk.

In fact, a well-known though ridiculed use of breast milk is against conjunctivitis. Fresh human milk instilled in the infected eyes is said to be effective against the conjunctival infection.

Anti-bodies against different types of bacteria, viruses, etc., have been found in the breast milk. They protect against all kinds of infection—from chest, ear, intestinal to skin infections.

The cells contained in milk are similar to the cells in blood.

Thus human milk is very much a "live milk" with unique anti-infective properties.

...and Allergies

Incidence of allergic disease increases if infant is not on human milk.

Most cases of allergy start within the first 1-2 months of life, in infants on cow's milk. Bottle-feeding is one cause.

Just as human milk protein is made up of different groups and sub-groups, so is cow's milk protein. These groups play a role in inducing allergy in human infants.

Anti-allergic properties of human milk is what protects the infant from a range of allergic conditions such as dermatitis, rhinitis, ear conditions, allergic diarrhoea, vomiting, etc.

Intake of human milk, especially colostrum, is the most important factor in the prevention of allergies in the infants. Breast-feeding should also be continued for 1½ to 2 years.

It should be remembered though that breast-feeding only minimises or prolongs the onset of allergy and does not completely eliminate it.

Perfect Nutrition

The unique composition of human milk providing proteins, fats, sugars, salts, water minerals, etc., proves perfect nutrition for the infant.

Every ingredient of human milk plays an important role in the infant's nutrition.

These nutritive properties of human milk are hard to substitute through formula feeds. Iron deficiency anaemia, protein energy malnutrition, kidney overload, vitamin deficiencies, calcium deficiency, etc., are prevented by breast-feeding.

An infant exclusively on human milk does not require supplementation of any sort for the initial 6 months.

Breast milk provides complete nutrition and more.

Money Saved is Money Earned!
You may be from a well off family, and can spend on bottles, teats, formulas, etc.

But have you thought of the huge medical bills you may incur?

You now know how cow's milk causes diseases.

You also know what harm bottle-feeding does.

So don't be surprised if your bottle fed child falls ill.

Also think of the time consumed in sterilising the bottle and the teats and preparing the formula.

By the way, when you buy the formula, the price includes that of packaging, advertising and marketing.

So why don't you spend some of that money on good food to enhance your milk production instead?

Mother-Child Bonding
Your child needs to be near you in its growing years.

The act of breast-feeding not only ensures physical proximity but also emotional bonding. This act goes a long way in strengthening mother-child ties.

Such closeness also helps to develop the infant's nervous system.

Bottle-feeding does not give the sense of security that breast-feeding does. Hence the need to breast-feed.

Prevent life threatening diseases
Did you know that breast-feeding helps you also?

You can prevent breast cancer, ovarian cancer, cancer of the uterus if you feed your baby.

You can also avoid obesity.

Osteoporosis or weakening of bones occurs in almost all menopausal women. You can slow down this process in late life if you breast-feed.

BIBLIOGRAPHY

1. Guyton A.C. - *Textbook of Medical Physiology*, W.B. Saunders. 1981. 1033-35.

2. Behrman Richard E. & Webb Kenneth H. - Nelson, *Textbook of Paediatrics*, (pocket companion) W.B. Saunders & Prism Books Pvt Ltd, India. 1993. 26-35; 69-70.

3. Satoskar R.S. & Bhandarkar S.D. - Satoskar, Kale, *Bhandarkar's Pharmacology and Pharmacotherapeutics*. Popular Prakashan, Bombay, 1985. 16-17; 395-399; 778-779; 797-798; 819-822; 853-860

4. Jellife D.D. & Jellife E.F.P. - *Human milk in the modern world*. English Language Society & Oxford University Press, 1977

5. Helsing Elizabeth & King F. Savage - *Breast-feeding in practice-A manual for health workers*. Delhi Oxford University Press 1984.

6. Percival Robert - Holland & Brews, *Manual of Obstetrics*. B. 1. Churchill Livingstone, 1986. 67-68; 120-122; 772-776.

7. Dr. (Mrs) Fernandez Armida & Stephen N. Monteiro - *Breast-feeding management - Steps towards Baby-Friendly Care*. UNICEF, Bombay.1994.

8. King F. Savage (Indian adaptation by Dr. Anand R.K.) - *Helping Mothers to Breast-feed*. ACASH Publication, 1994.